WHAT IS MENOPAUSE?

in the same series

What Is Pregnancy?
Kate E. Reynolds
Illustrated by Jonathon Powell
ISBN 978 1 78775 939 8
eISBN 978 1 78775 940 4

What Is Sex?
Kate E. Reynolds
Illustrated by Jonathon Powell
ISBN 978 1 78775 937 4
eISBN 978 1 78775 938 1

by the same author in the *Sexuality and Safety with Tom and Ellie* series

What's Happening to Ellie?
Kate E. Reynolds
Illustrated by Jonathon Powell
ISBN 978 1 84905 526 0
eISBN 978 0 85700 937 1

Things Ellie Likes
Kate E. Reynolds
Illustrated by Jonathon Powell
ISBN 978 1 84905 525 3
eISBN 978 0 85700 936 4

What's Happening to Tom?
Kate E. Reynolds
Illustrated by Jonathon Powell
ISBN 978 1 84905 523 9
eISBN 978 0 85700 934 0

Things Tom Likes
Kate E. Reynolds
Illustrated by Jonathon Powell
ISBN 978 1 84905 522 2
eISBN 978 0 85700 933 3

What Is Menopause?

A Guide for People with Autism, Special
Educational Needs and Disabilities

Kate E. Reynolds

Illustrated by Jonathon Powell

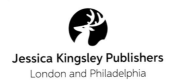

Jessica Kingsley Publishers
London and Philadelphia

First published in Great Britain in 2022 by Jessica Kingsley Publishers
An imprint of Hodder & Stoughton Ltd
An Hachette Company

1

A CIP catalogue record for this title is available from the British Library
and the Library of Congress

ISBN 978 1 78775 941 1
eISBN 978 1 78775 942 8

Printed and bound in China by Leo Paper Products

Jessica Kingsley Publishers' policy is to use papers that are natural, renewable
and recyclable products and made from wood grown in sustainable forests.
The logging and manufacturing processes are expected to conform to the
environmental regulations of the country of origin.

Jessica Kingsley Publishers
Carmelite House
50 Victoria Embankment
London EC4Y 0DZ

www.jkp.com

For Wendy Marilda (Thorogood) Garrad, with fond memories of interrailing across Europe, guided by her skilled use of the *Thomas Cook Overseas Timetable* book, and our tutor, Christopher Wilton Brown.

Kate

Thanks to all my friends and family, for their love, support and help through the years.

Jonathon

DISCLAIMER

Illustrations and wording in this book are explicit and the author and illustrator are not responsible for any offence that may be caused.

The content of this book should not be regarded as a substitute for the advice of a medical or mental health professional practitioner or recommended therapy, treatment or professional consultation. The author and illustrator are not responsible or liable for any diagnosis made or actions taken based on the content of this book. Always consult your family doctor or licensed mental health professional if you are concerned about your health or that of a person with autism or developmental and intellectual disabilities.

NOTES FOR FAMILIES AND SUPPORT STAFF

Menopause is rarely recognized or addressed with people who have autism, special educational needs and disabilities (SEND), yet it is a part of the life course which can be actively managed. Menopause affects women, transgender and non-binary people who have ovaries and uteruses.

Menopause significantly impacts daily living, so supporting people medically or through complementary therapies can fundamentally improve their lives. Families and support staff need a broad awareness of menopause to help individuals seek medical and complementary therapy to support them through what can be distressing years before and after menopause.

Symptoms related to dropping hormone levels are broad and vary from person to person. Doctors may take some time to accurately diagnose low hormone levels, and people with autism or SEND may need support and advocacy through this period.

Menopause is when someone has not had a period for 12 months, but the stages before menopause can take years and mark the end of fertility. Some people may never have known they could get pregnant, so this information may be upsetting to hear.

The average age of people in the UK to have menopause is 51 years, a time when their parents may die, which can intensify the effects of menopause, notably hormone-related depression.

As part of the *Healthy Loving, Healthy Living* series, this book uses explicit wording and illustrations and is gender-neutral. Each book can be read directly by individuals who have autism and SEND or with support.

If you have a womb, you are born with soft, tiny eggs in your ovaries. An egg can become a baby if it is fertilized by sperm during sex between a penis and a vagina. If your egg isn't fertilized, you have a period.

As you age, you release fewer eggs and your periods stop. People are about 45 years old when these changes start but can be younger or older. If you're under 40 years old and not having regular periods, check with your doctor that everything's okay.

Menopause is when you haven't had a period for 12 months. If you mark your periods on a calendar, you can work out when they're due and realize when they are stopping. The time before your periods stop completely is called perimenopause and can take months or years.

During perimenopause you might:

- Start losing more blood or less blood than usual during your period.
- Have fewer or irregular periods.
- Have a mix of heavy then light periods.

Not knowing when your period might happen can be distressing. It's a good idea to always carry sanitary supplies with you. If you have sensory issues, the feeling and smell of blood from your vagina can be challenging. Things that help you, like using tampons or changing your pad often, are really important in perimenopause.

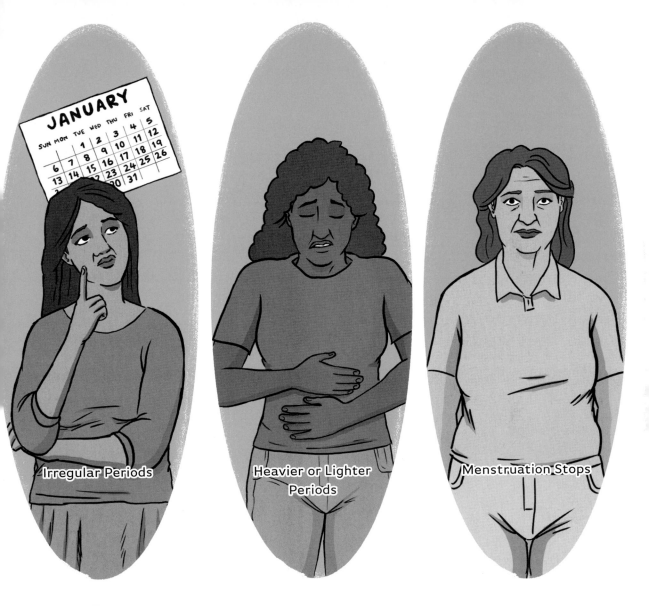

Irregular Periods

Heavier or Lighter Periods

Menstruation Stops

If you have a womb, you produce three important hormones, oestrogen, testosterone and progesterone, but you make less of these as you age. This can greatly affect your body and make you feel ill. You may have symptoms for up to 12 years before and after menopause.

- Oestrogen protects blood vessels in your heart, helps your brain and memory, keeps your bones strong, helps your mood and keeps areas of your body moist, like your bone joints, vagina, eyes and mouth.
- Testosterone keeps muscle bulk and helps with desire to have sex. It also gives energy and helps concentration.
- Progesterone helps with your periods and in pregnancy.

During puberty, your body became a different shape. As you get older, your body shape will change again.

Here are some of the changes you might see as you get older and hormone levels lower:

- Your arms and legs can look less muscly and the skin may hang down.
- Your jaw gets less clear and your neck skin sags.
- Your buttocks and belly may be less hard and start to droop down.
- The pubic hair on your vulva (the lips on the outside of your vagina), and head hair, can get thinner and turn grey.
- You put on weight, particularly around your waist.
- Your breasts droop more, look less round and are less firm with a wider gap between them.

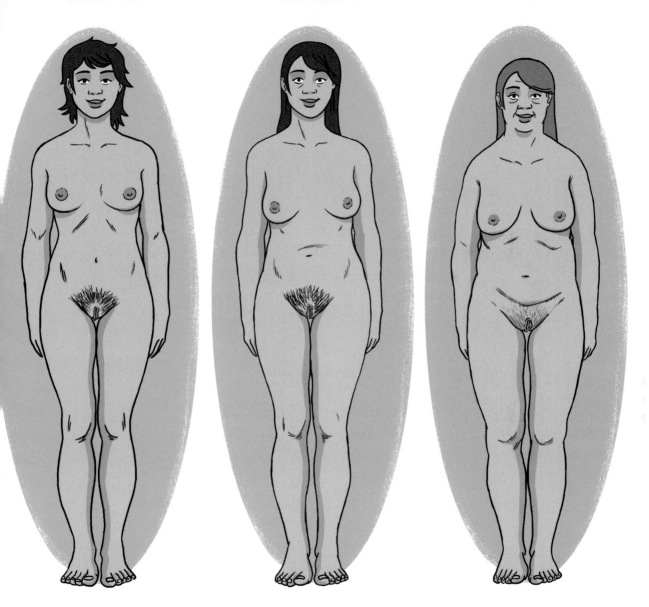

As you get older, you are more likely to get lumps in your breasts or in your armpits. Often these are harmless, like a cyst. However, sometimes lumps can be cancer.

It's very important to see your doctor if you find any lumps, however small or large. If you have breast cancer, the earlier you see a doctor, the more likely treatment will work. If you've had lumps before that weren't cancer, still report any new lumps to your doctor straight away.

Everyone's breasts are different, so it's important that you know your own breasts to spot any changes. Stand in front of a mirror with your hands on your hips and look for the following changes:

- Breast skin that is like orange peel or is swollen, red, darker than usual or bumpy.
- Breasts that look lop-sided or have changed shape.
- Nipples that have started to turn inwards or have sores, rashes, discharge or fluid.

Then look for the same things with your arms above your head. If you notice any changes, or have pain in any part of your breast or armpit, see your doctor.

As you get older, you have mammograms, which look for breast lumps and can find them before you can feel or see them. Your naked breasts are x-rayed by being squeezed between two metal plates. You have to stay very still. The squeezing can be uncomfortable but that should stop once the mammogram has finished.

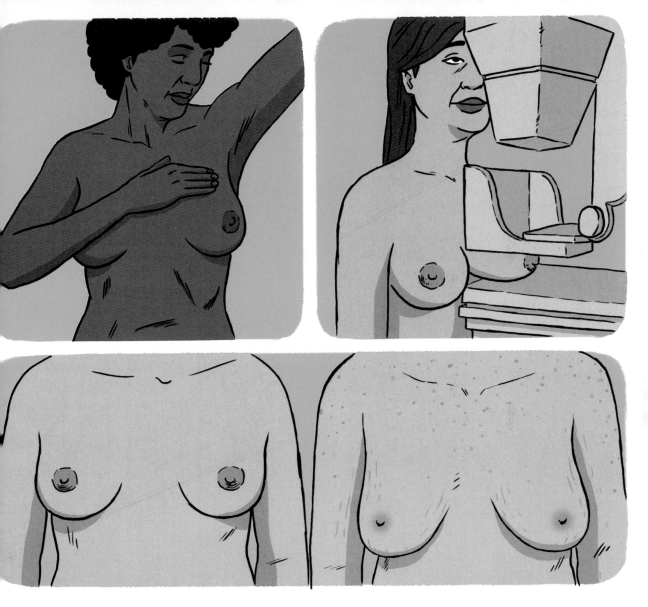

Hot flushes or hot flashes are common symptoms of dropping hormones. They make you suddenly hot and sweaty, and you can feel dizzy. This can happen many times a day, or as night sweats.

Night sweats may make your bed so wet that you have to change your sheets or clothes. You might find it hard to go back to sleep as your body cools down.

If you get hot flushes or hot flashes, these things might help you:

- Wear clothes that aren't heavy and are cool, like loose cotton shirts.
- Have layers that you can take off easily, like a cardigan on top of a t-shirt.
- Have a cool shower or bath, use a fan and have cold drinks.
- Keep your bedroom cool overnight. If it's safe, open your windows, use a fan or air conditioning.
- Avoid spicy foods, coffee, smoking and alcohol.
- Exercise regularly and keep a healthy weight.
- Keep anxiety levels low.

Hot flushes or hot flashes can make you feel out of control and uncertain, which makes you anxious. Being wet and feeling cold can be particularly distressing if you have sensory issues. Disturbances in your sleep can make you feel tired and grumpy and crave sweet foods during the day.

It's important to talk about hot flushes or flashes and night sweats with your doctor to make sure it is low hormones causing them and get medicine to help.

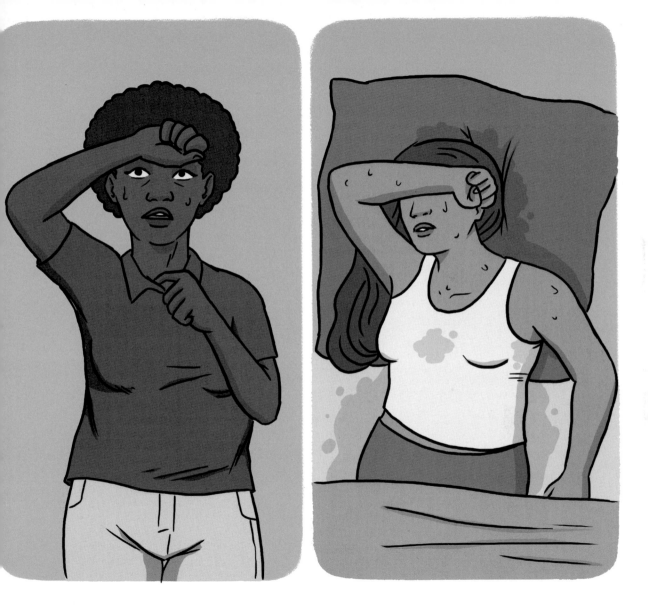

Low hormone levels affect how you feel about things (your mood). You may find you have changes in your mood which are hard to control. This is more likely if you get premenstrual syndrome (when, for example, you have mood swings, anxiety, a bloated belly and painful breasts before a period) or had postnatal depression if you had a baby. These things show that your body is sensitive to changes in your hormones.

Changes in mood can include any of these:

- Feeling anxious or worried all the time.
- Feeling angry or annoyed without knowing why.
- Feeling irritated by things or getting frustrated with things.
- Having panic attacks and anxiety, which can be distressing and hard to control.
- Feeling very low or sad or wanting to cry without knowing why. You may not have had any depression in your life before, so this can be hard to manage.

Your doctor may prescribe hormone replacement therapy (HRT) instead of antidepressants because it's your low hormones that are causing your low mood. If you can't take HRT for a medical reason, you may be given antidepressants.

Some foods can make your mood better, such as eggs or oily fish like mackerel, salmon, sardines and anchovies. Other foods like dairy (milk, cheese), nuts, seeds, green vegetables, meats and chicken also help with mood.

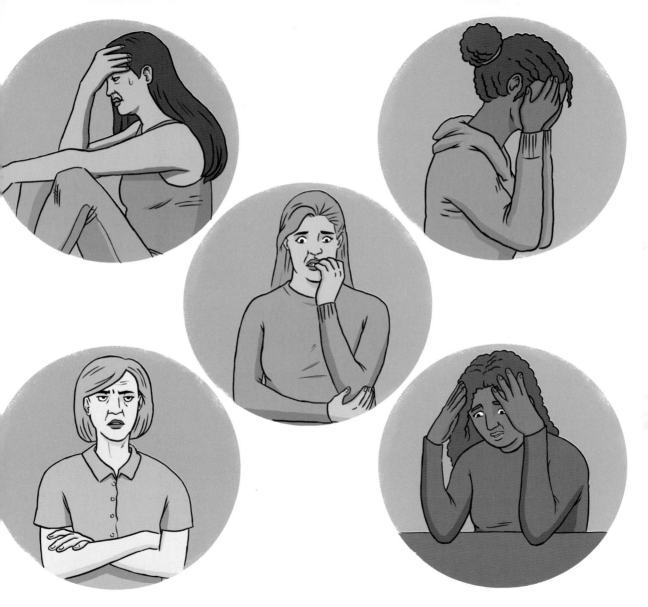

Hormones help your brain work properly, so dropping hormone levels can affect your brain in many ways. Low hormone levels might mean you have:

- Problems remembering things or being unable to concentrate on things you could before.
- Headaches.
- "Brain fog" when it's difficult to do ordinary thinking that you could do before. Some people think they have dementia because they can't think straight. This foggy thinking can cause you to have a low mood.
- Difficulty getting to sleep, often caused by high levels of anxiety. You might also wake up a lot in the night, even if you don't have night sweats. This is particularly caused by low progesterone and testosterone.

- Poor sleep, which can affect how your day goes if you feel constantly exhausted, which means you can't think clearly.

Linked to these brain effects are effects on your nervous system, which can cause numbness or a burning or itching feeling in your hands and feet. This can make getting to sleep difficult and can wake you as well.

You can help yourself by eating well, not drinking alcohol or smoking, limiting caffeine (which is found in coffee, tea and some cold drinks) and getting regular exercise. You should always report these symptoms to your doctor to make sure they are from low hormones, not other illnesses, and to get treatment.

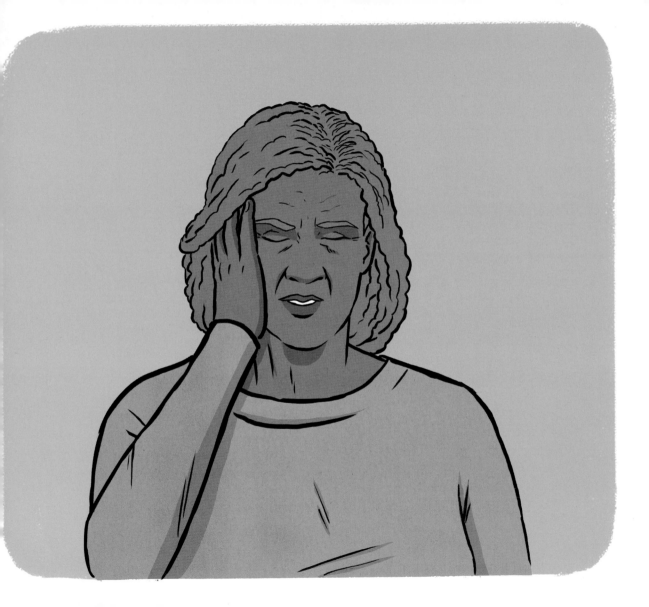

Oestrogen helps keep fluid in your joints so they move easily. As your hormones lower, the fluid dries up, so your joints become stiff and painful. Your hips and knees may hurt most, because they carry your weight. As testosterone drops, the amount of muscle in your body shrinks, so you're not as strong.

Things that make joint pain worse:

- Hormones decrease: HRT is explained later and helps by replacing low hormones.
- Dehydration: This is when your body doesn't have enough fluid. You can lose fluid from night or day sweats, by drinking too little and drinking alcohol. Check with your doctor and try to drink 1–2 litres of water every day and limit alcohol.

- Gaining weight: Because of changes in your body and being less active, you may gain weight. You might feel tired and anxious, which often causes people to eat sugary and high-fat foods leading to weight gain.
- Poor posture: You may start to sit or stand poorly to take pressure off a painful joint, but this can strain and hurt other joints.

Things that can help:

- Swimming, cycling and walking are gentle on joints and build strength. Stretching and warm baths help with stiff joints.
- Doctors can check you don't have arthritis, which needs different treatment. They can also refer you to a chiropractor or osteopath, who specialize in bone health.

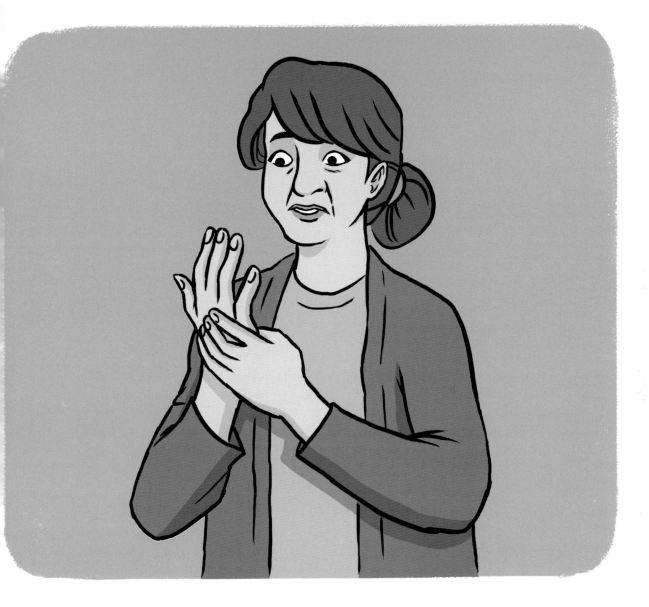

When oestrogen lowers, bones grow less quickly and can break easily. Over time, you might develop osteoporosis. Osteoporosis causes your spine (back bone) to bend. There are treatments but these things make you more likely to get osteoporosis:

- Osteoporosis is in your family.
- Taking steroids for a long time or in high doses for conditions like asthma or arthritis.
- Eating disorders, such as anorexia, bulimia or compulsive eating.
- Medical conditions, such as coeliac or Crohn's diseases of the bowel.
- Heavy drinking of alcohol or smoking.
- Taking breast cancer medication that reduces hormone levels quickly.
- Not being active or having to stay in bed for long periods of time.

How to prevent osteoporosis:

- Exercise regularly, especially doing weight-bearing exercises, like walking, and resistance exercises, like weight training.
- Stop smoking and cut down or cut out alcohol.
- Eat healthily, with fresh fruit, vegetables, pulses (like chickpeas and lentils) and beans. Also eat foods containing calcium, such as milk and cheeses. If you're vegan, try alternative milks and cheeses. Limit very processed foods and keep sugar and salt to a minimum.
- Take HRT if prescribed.
- Get sunlight (but don't sunbathe without sun block or use sunbeds). This helps your body produce vitamin D which keeps your bones strong. Vitamin D can also be prescribed by your doctor.

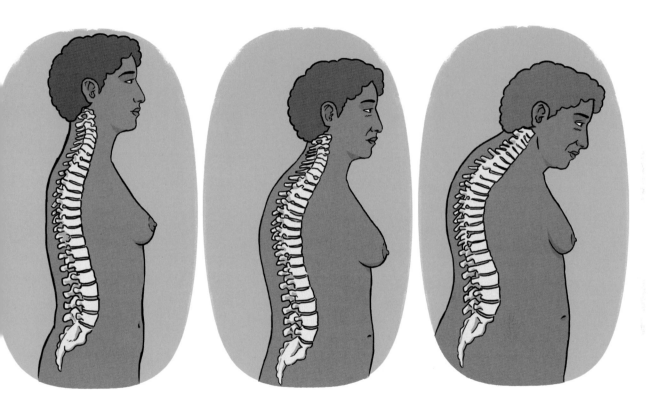

Oestrogen keeps your vagina and vulva moist, and without it the walls of your vagina get thinner, drier and less stretchy. Your vagina and skin nearby can feel sore and itchy. This can make it difficult to concentrate and to sit down.

You can also get Thrush, which is a fungal infection of your vagina and vulva. This causes thick, creamy discharge and small white patches that itch. It can be particularly painful when you're using tampons or when you're having sex.

Your bladder (which contains your pee in your body) and the tube from the bladder to the outside (which you pee through) also get thinner without oestrogen. This can make you pee more often and more urgently. You might get more urine infections and leak pee when you sneeze, cough or laugh.

Your doctor can prescribe ways to treat vaginal dryness, such as:

- Oestrogen cream to put on your vagina and vulva.
- A pessary, which is a small tablet that you put inside your vagina using your fingers or an applicator, like inserting a tampon.
- An oestrogen ring. This is explained later.

If you can't take oestrogen, you can use non-hormonal moisturizers on your vulva and inside your vagina. If you're going to have sex, you should use water-based lubricants which don't damage condoms. Moisturizers and lubricants can both be bought at pharmacies.

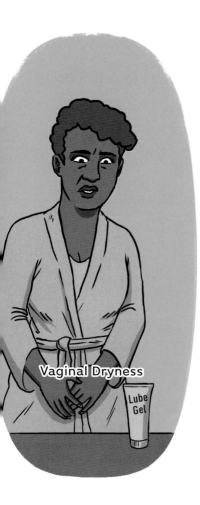

Vaginal Dryness

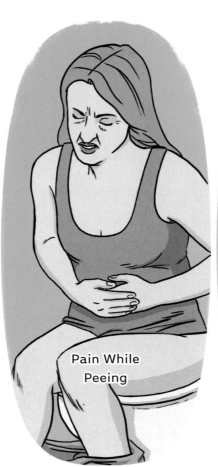

Pain While
Peeing

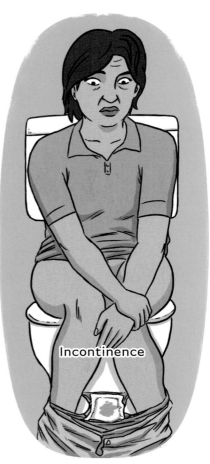

Incontinence

Losing hormones can affect your intimate relationships. There are lots of reasons for this:

- You may lose interest in lots of things, including sex.
- Your vagina may be dry and itchy, which can make having sex uncomfortable or painful.
- You may not feel good about yourself, because your energy levels are low, your hair can become thin and you might put on weight.
- You may have difficulty controlling your mood, which can affect how well you and your partner get on.

Masturbation (touching yourself for pleasure) can make your vulva sore due to rubbing. Vaginal cream or water-based lubricant can relieve this.

HRT may help with these symptoms. Some people think that HRT is the same as being on a contraceptive pill. HRT does contain the same kind of hormones but in much smaller amounts. So, there are some important things to know:

- If you're still having periods and taking HRT, you can get pregnant, so you should always use contraception, like condoms.
- You need to check with your doctor but generally, if you're under 50 years old, you can stop using contraception after two years without a period. Once you're 55 years old, it's thought that you can't get pregnant naturally.

Your doctor may refer you for couple counselling to support your relationship.

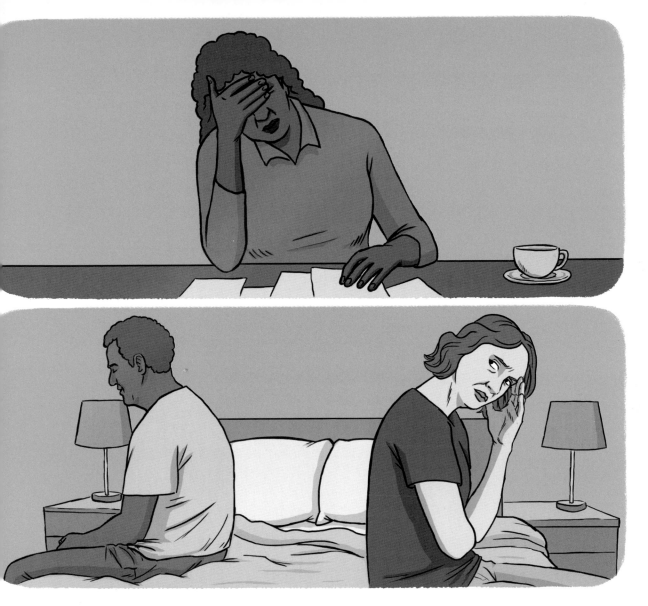

Oestrogen protects your blood vessels (the arteries and veins that lead to and from your heart), so lower hormones can affect the blood system in your body.

In the short term, you may have palpitations, which is when your heart suddenly beats quickly and you notice the pounding. This can make you feel dizzy, out of control and distressed. This often happens at the same time as hot flushes or hot flashes.

Over years, fatty bits can build up in your blood vessels and cause a greater risk of blood clots, which can cause heart attacks or strokes. Fatty build-up can also cause dementia and affect your kidneys.

Oestrogen helps keep your blood sugar steady. Without it, you are more likely to get type 2 diabetes. This is when your blood sugar isn't controlled and affects your blood vessels, heart and the flow of blood around your body.

HRT can reduce the damage from low hormones. It doesn't matter if you're still having periods or if you've had your menopause recently or even years before, HRT can still work.

You can help prevent heart disease by not smoking, limiting alcohol, getting regular exercise and eating lots of fruits and vegetables.

Also, limit highly processed foods, which contain chemicals, flavourings, colourings and sweeteners, such as fizzy drinks, salty snacks, some breakfast cereals, pre-prepared (ready) meals, sausages and candy.

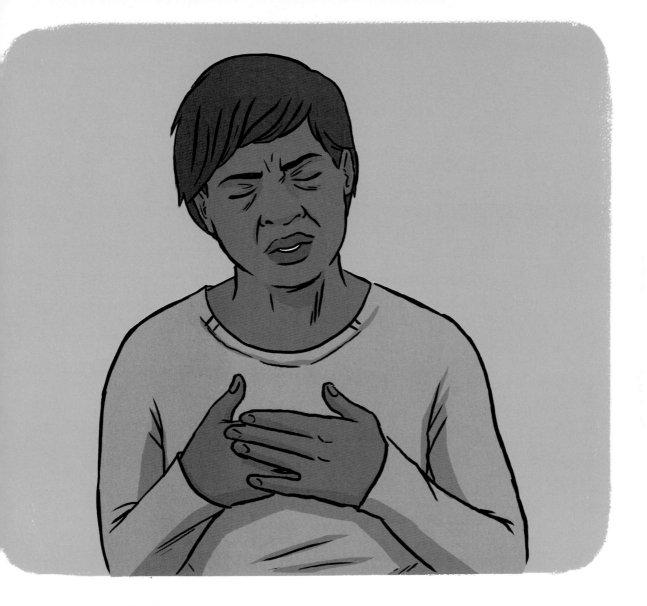

It's important to get medical help with symptoms. Your doctor can work out if your symptoms are due to lower hormones or another condition.

Your doctor can prescribe HRT which contains hormones to replace the ones that have dropped. You can start taking HRT when you're still having periods. After you start taking HRT, it can take up to three months for your symptoms to improve. You should let your doctor know if you don't feel better.

HRT can help with lots of symptoms which affect your brain, your vagina and urinary systems, your muscles and joints, and your energy levels. It also helps prevent osteoporosis and heart disease.

HRT can be given in these ways:

- Tablets or pills.
- Skin patches, like a plaster put onto the skin of the leg, upper arm or other places advised on the information in the package.
- Gel to rub into your skin, usually onto your inner thighs or other places as advised on the information in the package.

Your doctor won't prescribe HRT if you've had breast, ovarian or womb cancers. This is because these cancers are treated with medication that lowers hormones, rather than raises them.

Research used to show that HRT was linked to breast cancer. Today, medicines in HRT are different and doctors can work out what's best on an individual basis.

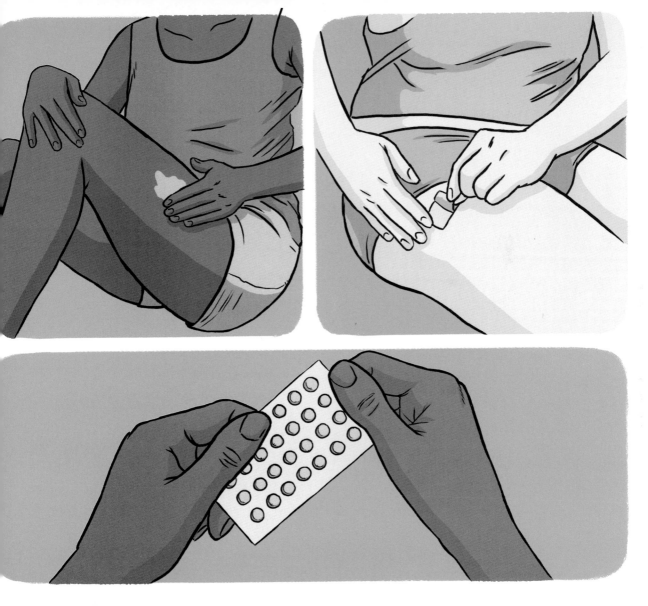

HRT treatments include:

- A vaginal hormone ring. This is a soft, bendy ring made of silicon, placed in the vagina. If you have sensory issues, you may find feeling inside your vagina distressing.

  A health professional can insert the ring for you, if you find it difficult. Once in place, the ring gives out a low, steady dose of oestrogen. After three months it can be replaced. You can have sex with the ring in, but if it's uncomfortable, it's possible to remove it, clean it, then put it back in after sex.

- An implant (like a tablet) under your skin, often in the abdomen (belly) or the buttocks (bottom). The implant is put inside in a sterile way and the doctor will numb your skin to prevent pain.

Some people prefer having the implant in their buttocks so they can't see the procedure. The implant stays inside you, giving off hormones for several months. After this, your symptoms may start to return. Your doctor will give you a blood test before a new implant is inserted.

Medication prescribed for other conditions, such as Gabapentin (epilepsy) and Clonidine (high blood pressure), can help manage low hormones. Sometimes, antidepressants are given to reduce day and night sweats. All of these medications can reduce anxiety and vaginal dryness too.

Tell your doctor if you have vaginal bleeding, discharge or discomfort.

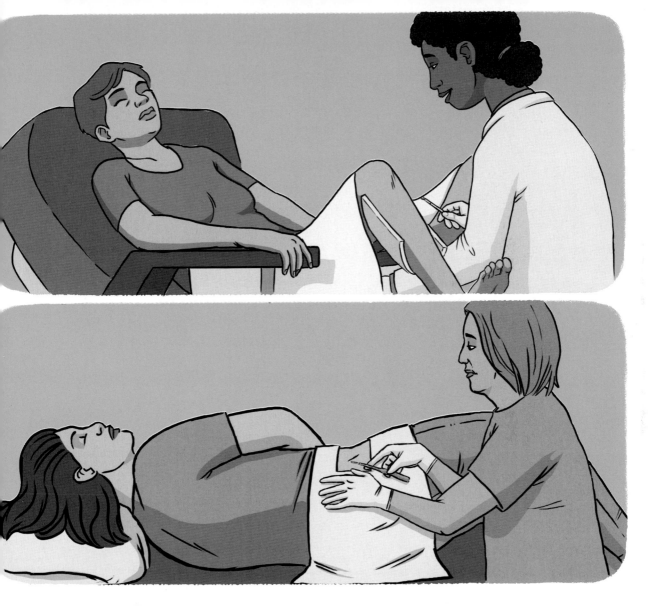

There are other things you can do, including trying complementary therapies. It's important to tell your doctor what you're doing, to make sure it doesn't affect any medications prescribed for you.

- Regular exercise, for example, swimming, brisk walking or an exercise class for 30 minutes a few times a week, keeps muscles strong and weight under control and helps reduce anxiety.
- Herbal medicines, such as black cohosh, which is sold to help with menopause and osteoporosis. While herbal medicines may seem safe because they're natural, when mixed with certain prescribed medicines, they can make you ill, so it's really important to discuss them with your doctor.
- Cognitive behavioural therapy (CBT) can help with depression and anxiety. You can talk to a counsellor and they will help you develop skills to deal with challenges. Your doctor can refer you to a counsellor or you can look for one privately, but make sure they are a member of a national or state agency.
- Yoga and meditation can help with managing thoughts and with relaxation. Yoga also strengthens bones and muscles.
- Several therapies help reduce anxiety. These include aromatherapy, where fragrances are used with massage to help you relax, and acupuncture, where tiny needles are put into your skin. These therapies may not be possible if you have sensory issues.

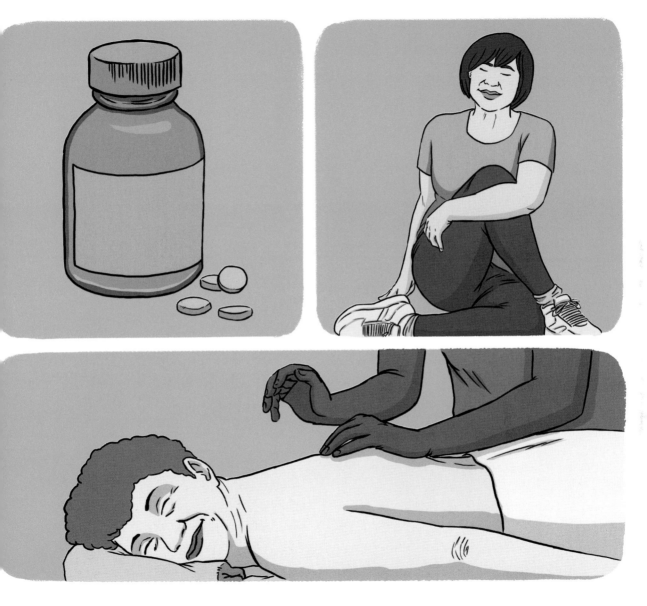

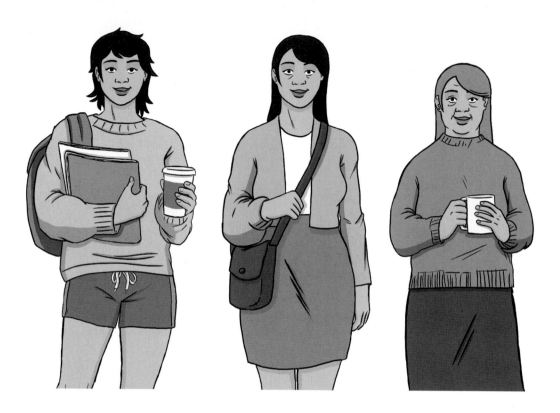

Although losing hormones can affect all parts of your body in different ways, there are many things you can do to feel better. The most important thing is to make sure you see a doctor. Ensure you have a trusted person with you or an advocate if you need one. If your symptoms don't get better, keep going back to the doctor. Eat healthily, don't smoke or drink too much alcohol, take regular exercise – and enjoy life!

HOW TO CHECK YOUR BREASTS

Remember to look in the mirror at your breasts (see page 12).

Lie down and feel your naked breasts. Start by using one hand to feel the breast on the other side of your body. Put your fingers together to make a pad then press down so that you squash your breast between your fingers and your ribs below. Move your fingers around in small circles. Start feeling your nipple and move outwards. Get to know what your breasts feel like usually.

Areas to cover: top to bottom of your breast, from your collar bone (the bone at the top of your chest) to the top of your abdomen (belly). Then side to side, covering from your armpit to your cleavage (the space between your breasts).

After going through the process lying down, do the same thing sitting or standing up. Some people find it easier to examine their breasts with wet hands, so you can also do this in the bath or shower.

HOW TO MAKE A DOCTOR'S APPOINTMENT

- Have your diary ready or write down dates when you're free in the next few weeks to have an appointment. Write down your cell phone or mobile number because the service may ask for this so they can text you with your appointment details.
- When you ring the service, tell the person speaking to you what difference you have, like a learning disability or autism. This helps the person support you to understand and to give you more time if you want it.
- Ask for a double appointment slot if you have processing difficulties and it takes you a long time to understand information.
- Write down why you need an appointment, like "I have symptoms of menopause". You may want a woman or man doctor, so you can say that. You don't have to tell anyone why you want an appointment, but it can help the person to work out how quickly to get your appointment.
- Write the appointment date and time down immediately and repeat it back to the person on the phone so you get it right.

WHAT TO SAY IN AN APPOINTMENT

It's a good idea to take someone with you for support. Write down a list of symptoms and how often you get them. You can work this out over a two-week period then give it to the doctor to see.

Also write a list of any herbal medicines or other supplements you're taking, so the doctor can take these into account if they prescribe you any medicine.

Symptoms

- Change in periods
- Hot flushes or hot flashes
- Changes in moods
- Joint aches and pains
- Dry vagina
- Sore vulva
- Thrush infection
- Lack of sex drive
- Poor memory
- Dizziness
- Putting on weight
- Dry eyes
- Dry mouth and tongue
- Loss of interest in anything
- Depression
- Leaking pee
- Palpitations
- Night sweats
- Difficulty sleeping
- Low energy
- Thinning hair
- Cystitis (pee infection)
- Feeling anxious
- Sore gums
- Panic attacks
- Brain fog
- Numbness (pins and needles)
- Other _____

Kate E. Reynolds, MDS, PGDC, PGDHE, BSc (Hons) SA, RGN, is a mother to two children on the autism spectrum, one of whom has intellectual disabilities. She worked for the UK's National Health Service for 18 years, much of which was in HIV and sexual health. Kate has written 12 books, most published by Jessica Kingsley Publishers and almost all about aspects of relationships and sexuality. She works closely with parents, caregivers and health educators, as a public speaker, trainer, advisor and researcher.

Kate can be accessed through her websites at **www.kateereynolds.com** or **www.autismagonyaunt.com**

Jonathon Powell lives in Brisbane, Australia and has a Diploma in Fine Art and Bachelor of Animation from Griffith University, Queensland. He has illustrated for the *Sexuality and Safety with Tom and Ellie* six-book series by Kate E. Reynolds, *Can I tell you about Pathological Demand Avoidance syndrome?* by Ruth Fidler and Phil Christie, and *Making Sense of Sex* by Sarah Attwood, all published by Jessica Kingsley Publishers. He provided artwork and animations for Family Planning Queensland. Jonathon also illustrated *What are... Relationships?* by Kate E. Reynolds.